Chair Yoga Simple Guide for Beginners

Understanding the Importance of Chair Yoga

By

Greig Keaton

Table of Contents

CHAPTER 1

Introduction

Chair Yoga is a gentle and accessible form of yoga that has gained popularity in recent years for its inclusivity and adaptability. we will explore what Chair Yoga is, delve into the numerous benefits it offers, and examine the diverse range of individuals who can benefit from this practice.

1.1 What is Chair Yoga

Chair Yoga is a modified form of traditional yoga that is designed to be practiced while seated on a chair or with the support of a chair for balance and stability. It combines the fundamental principles of yoga, such as breathing, stretching, and meditation, with the convenience of a chair as a prop. Chair Yoga makes yoga accessible to a wider audience, including those who may have physical limitations or difficulty with traditional yoga poses.

In Chair Yoga, practitioners perform a series of gentle and controlled movements that help improve flexibility, strength, balance, and relaxation. These movements are adapted to accommodate various physical abilities and can be easily customized to suit individual needs. Chair Yoga is not only practiced in a seated position but can also incorporate standing and balancing poses with the aid of the chair.

The essence of Chair Yoga lies in making the healing and

transformative benefits of yoga accessible to everyone, regardless of age, mobility, or fitness level. It can be practiced by seniors, people with disabilities, individuals recovering from injuries, office workers, and anyone looking for a more accessible approach to yoga.

1.2 Benefits of Chair Yoga

Chair Yoga offers a wide range of physical, mental, and emotional benefits. Some of the key advantages include:

1. **Improved Flexibility:** Chair Yoga helps increase joint mobility and flexibility, making daily movements easier and reducing the risk of injury.

2. **Enhanced Strength:** The gentle resistance provided by Chair Yoga movements helps strengthen muscles, especially in the upper body and core.

3. **Better Posture:** Practicing Chair Yoga encourages proper alignment and awareness of posture, which can alleviate chronic back and neck pain.

4. **Stress Reduction:** Chair Yoga incorporates deep breathing and relaxation techniques, promoting stress relief and mental calmness.

5. **Increased Circulation:** The gentle movements stimulate blood flow, which can benefit heart health and reduce the risk of blood clots.

6. **Enhanced Balance:** Chair Yoga includes balancing poses that help improve stability and reduce the risk of falls, especially for seniors.

7. **Pain Management:** It can be used as a complementary therapy for managing chronic pain conditions like arthritis and fibromyalgia.

8. **Mind-Body Connection:** Chair Yoga emphasizes mindfulness and meditation, fostering a stronger connection between the mind and body.

9. **Accessibility:** Chair Yoga makes yoga accessible to those with physical limitations, allowing them to experience the benefits of yoga practice.

10. **Community and Social Interaction:** Chair Yoga classes provide a sense of community and social interaction, reducing feelings of isolation.

1.3 Who Can Benefit from Chair Yoga

Chair Yoga is a practice that extends its benefits to a wide range of individuals, making it an inclusive and welcoming form of exercise and mindfulness. Here are some of the groups of people who can benefit from Chair Yoga:

1. **Seniors:** Chair Yoga is gentle on the joints and can help seniors maintain or improve

their mobility, flexibility, and balance as they age.

2. **Individuals with Mobility Issues:** People with mobility limitations, whether due to injury, illness, or disability, can practice Chair Yoga to improve their physical well-being.

3. **Office Workers:** Those who spend long hours sitting at a desk can use Chair Yoga to relieve tension, reduce stress, and counteract the negative effects of prolonged sitting.

4. **Rehabilitation Patients:** Chair Yoga can be a valuable part of rehabilitation programs, aiding in the recovery process from injuries or surgeries.

5. **Stress Management:** Anyone looking for stress relief,

relaxation, and improved mental well-being can benefit from the mindfulness and meditation aspects of Chair Yoga.

6. **Pregnant Individuals:** Chair Yoga can be adapted for pregnant individuals to promote comfort and relaxation during pregnancy.

7. **Caregivers:** Chair Yoga offers caregivers a convenient way to manage their own physical and mental well-being, which is essential for their ability to provide care effectively.

8. **Those New to Yoga:** Chair Yoga provides an excellent introduction to yoga for beginners who may be

intimidated by more strenuous forms of practice.

Chair Yoga is a versatile and inclusive practice that can benefit individuals of all ages and physical abilities. Its adaptability and focus on gentle movements, mindfulness, and relaxation make it a valuable tool for improving overall well-being and promoting a healthier, more balanced lifestyle. Whether you're seeking physical fitness, stress relief, or a greater mind-body connection, Chair Yoga offers something for everyone.

CHAPTER 2

Getting Started with Chair Yoga

Chair Yoga is an accessible and versatile practice, but before you dive in, it's essential to get started on the right foot. In this section, we'll explore the key considerations for beginning your Chair Yoga journey, including selecting the appropriate chair, ensuring comfort and safety, and preparing the necessary clothing and equipment.

2.1 Choosing the Right Chair

Selecting the right chair is crucial for a comfortable and effective Chair Yoga practice. Here are some guidelines for choosing the appropriate chair:

1. **Sturdy and Stable:** Ensure that the chair you use is sturdy and stable, with no wobbling or loose parts. It should provide solid support during your practice.

2. **Armless or with Armrests:** While armless chairs are ideal for a broader range of movements, chairs with armrests can also be used, depending on your comfort and specific needs. Armrests can

provide extra support during seated poses.

3. **Comfortable Seat:** Look for a chair with a cushioned and comfortable seat. You'll be spending time sitting in it, so comfort is essential.

4. **No Wheels:** Avoid using chairs with wheels as they may roll unexpectedly during your practice, posing a safety risk.

5. **Proper Height:** The chair should allow your feet to rest flat on the floor with your knees at a 90-degree angle. This position promotes stability and proper alignment.

6. **Back Support:** Ensure the chair has a supportive backrest, especially if you plan to do

standing poses with chair
support.

7. **No Slip Covers:** Avoid chairs
   with slippery or loose-fitting
   covers that might cause you to
   slide during your practice.

2.2 Comfort and Safety Precautions

Safety and comfort are paramount in
Chair Yoga. Here are some
precautions to keep in mind:

1. **Clear Space:** Practice in a
   clear, uncluttered area to
   prevent tripping or bumping
   into objects while moving on
   and off the chair.

2. **Secure Chair Position:** Place
   the chair on a non-slip surface

and make sure it doesn't slide or
move during your practice.

3. **Maintain Proper Alignment:**
   Pay close attention to your
   posture and alignment, ensuring
   that you sit upright with your
   feet flat on the floor.

4. **Listen to Your Body:** Respect
   your body's limits and avoid
   pushing yourself too hard.
   Chair Yoga is meant to be
   gentle and should not cause
   discomfort or pain.

5. **Use Props as Needed:**
   Depending on your flexibility
   and mobility, you may use
   additional props like cushions
   or blocks to support your
   practice and maintain comfort.

6. **Stay Hydrated:** Like any
   physical activity, Chair Yoga

may cause you to perspire. Stay
hydrated by having water
nearby.

2.3 Clothing and Equipment

Proper clothing and equipment can enhance your Chair Yoga experience:

1. **Comfortable Clothing:** Wear loose, comfortable clothing that allows for a full range of motion. Avoid clothes that are too tight or restrictive.

2. **Footwear:** In most Chair Yoga practices, you'll be barefoot or wearing non-slip socks. This allows for better stability and grip on the floor.

3. **Mat or Non-Slip Surface:**
    Placing a yoga mat or a non-slip surface under the chair can improve stability and reduce the risk of the chair sliding.

4. **Props:** Depending on your practice, you may use props like yoga blocks, cushions, or resistance bands to enhance your experience and adapt poses to your needs.

5. **Water Bottle:** Keep a water bottle nearby to stay hydrated throughout your practice.

Carefully considering these factors when getting started with Chair Yoga, you can create a safe and comfortable environment for your practice. This will allow you to focus on the many physical and mental benefits that Chair Yoga has to offer.

CHAPTER 3

Basic Chair Yoga Poses

Chair Yoga offers a variety of poses that can be adapted to accommodate different levels of mobility and flexibility.

3.1 Seated Mountain Pose

Seated Mountain Pose is the foundation of many Chair Yoga sequences, and it serves as a starting point for centering and grounding yourself. Here's how to do it:

1. Begin by sitting comfortably on your chair with your feet flat on the floor and your knees aligned with your hips.

2. Rest your hands on your thighs, palms facing down.

3. Lengthen your spine, imagining it reaching toward the ceiling, and engage your core muscles gently.

4. Relax your shoulders away from your ears, keeping them down and back.

5. Close your eyes if comfortable and focus on your breath. Inhale deeply through your nose and exhale through your mouth, maintaining a sense of stability and balance.

6. Hold this pose for a few deep breaths, feeling grounded and centered.

Seated Mountain Pose is an excellent starting point for any Chair Yoga practice, helping you establish a strong foundation and mindfulness.

3.2 Seated Forward Bend

The *Seated Forward Bend* is a gentle stretch that can help release tension in the back and hamstrings. Here's how to perform it:

1. Begin in a seated position, as in Seated Mountain Pose.

2. Inhale, lengthening your spine and sitting tall.

3. As you exhale, hinge at your hips and slowly begin to lean

forward. Keep your back straight and maintain a gentle curve in your lower back.

4. Extend your arms toward your feet, reaching for your shins, ankles, or the floor, depending on your flexibility. If you can't reach your feet, simply reach as far as is comfortable.

5. Breathe deeply and relax into the stretch. Feel the gentle pull along your back and the back of your legs.

6. Hold this pose for several breaths, gradually deepening the stretch with each exhale.

7. To come out of the pose, inhale and slowly sit back up, stacking your spine one vertebra at a time.

Seated Forward Bend is an excellent pose for relieving tension in the lower back and improving flexibility in the hamstrings.

3.3 Seated Twist

The *Seated Twist* is a pose that helps improve spinal mobility and promotes digestion. Here's how to do it:

1. Begin in your seated position, ensuring your feet are flat on the floor and your spine is tall.

2. Inhale, lengthening your spine.

3. Exhale as you gently twist your upper body to the right. Place your left hand on the outside of your right thigh and your right hand on the back of the chair, near your lower back.

4. Keep your hips square and avoid twisting at the waist. Focus on twisting from your mid to upper back.

5. Inhale to lengthen your spine even more, and exhale to deepen the twist slightly. Look over your right shoulder if it's comfortable for your neck.

6. Hold the twist for a few breaths, feeling the stretch along your spine.

7. Inhale to come back to the center and exhale as you repeat the twist to the left side.

8. Hold the twist on the left side for the same duration.

Seated Twist is a beneficial pose for maintaining spinal health and can provide relief from tension and stiffness in the back.

These basic Chair Yoga poses are a great starting point for building strength, flexibility, and mindfulness while seated comfortably in a chair. As you become more familiar with these poses, you can incorporate them into longer Chair Yoga sequences for a well-rounded practice.

3.4 Seated Cat-Cow Stretch

The *Seated Cat-Cow Stretch* is a gentle sequence that helps increase spinal flexibility and release tension in the back. Here's how to perform it:

1. Begin in your seated position with feet flat on the floor, maintaining a tall spine.

2. Inhale as you arch your back, lifting your chest and drawing your shoulder blades together. This is the Cow position.

3. Exhale as you round your back, tucking your chin toward your chest and bringing your navel toward your spine. This is the Cat position.

4. Continue to flow between the Cow and Cat positions with your breath. Inhale for Cow, and exhale for Cat.

5. Repeat this gentle rocking motion for several breaths, allowing the movement to flow smoothly.

6. This stretch helps improve spinal mobility, increases awareness of your breath, and

releases tension in the back and
shoulders.

3.5 Seated Warrior Pose

Seated Warrior Pose is a variation of
the classic Warrior Pose from
traditional yoga. It helps strengthen
your core and improve balance while
seated in a chair:

1. Begin in your seated position
   with feet flat on the floor and a
   tall spine.

2. Inhale as you reach your arms
   overhead, stretching them
   upward.

3. Exhale as you bend your right
   elbow and bring your right
   hand behind your head, palm
   facing your upper back.

4. Inhale again, extending your left arm out to the side, palm facing down.

5. Exhale and lean to the right, keeping your left hand reaching to the side, creating a side stretch in your torso.

6. Hold the stretch for a few breaths, feeling the stretch along your left side.

7. Inhale to return to an upright position, and then exhale to repeat the stretch on the left side.

8. Hold the stretch on the left side for the same duration.

Seated Warrior Pose is an excellent way to work on balance and strengthen your core muscles while seated in a chair, promoting stability and flexibility.

3.6 Seated Tree Pose

Seated Tree Pose is a chair adaptation of the traditional Tree Pose in yoga, focusing on balance and leg strength. Here's how to do it:

1. Begin in your seated position with feet flat on the floor, maintaining an upright posture.

2. Place your right foot on the inside of your left calf, just above the ankle. Your right knee should be pointing out to the side.

3. Find your balance, and if you're comfortable, bring your hands to your heart center in a prayer position.

4. Hold this pose for several breaths, focusing on your balance and stability.

5. Release your right foot and return it to the floor.

6. Repeat the same sequence on the other side, placing your left foot on the inside of your right calf.

7. Hold the pose for the same duration on the left side.

Seated Tree Pose challenges your balance and strengthens your leg muscles while providing a sense of grounding and stability. It can be adapted to your level of flexibility and balance.

These Chair Yoga poses, including the Seated Cat-Cow Stretch, Seated Warrior Pose, and Seated Tree Pose, add variety and depth to your practice, targeting different areas of the body and offering a range of physical and mental benefits. Incorporate them into your Chair Yoga routine to continue improving your flexibility, strength, and overall well-being while seated comfortably in a chair.

CHAPTER 4

Chair Yoga Sequences

Chair Yoga sequences are a structured way to incorporate a series of poses and movements into your practice, offering specific benefits depending on the sequence's focus.

4.1 Morning Chair Yoga Sequence

This Chair Yoga sequence is designed to invigorate your body and mind, setting a positive tone for the day ahead. It focuses on gentle stretches and movements to wake up your muscles and increase circulation.

1. **Seated Mountain Pose (Centering):** Start your morning Chair Yoga session with Seated Mountain Pose to center yourself. Sit with your feet flat on the floor, hands on your thighs, and focus on deep, mindful breaths for a few moments.

2. **Seated Cat-Cow Stretch:** Move into the Seated Cat-Cow Stretch to awaken your spine and relieve stiffness. Flow between these two poses for a minute, inhaling for Cow and exhaling for Cat.

3. **Seated Forward Bend:** Perform the Seated Forward Bend to stretch your hamstrings and lower back. Hold the pose for five deep breaths, gradually reaching toward your feet.

4. **Seated Side Stretch:** Sit up tall and inhale as you lift your right arm overhead, exhaling as you bend to the left, creating a gentle side stretch. Hold for a few breaths and repeat on the other side.

5. **Seated Twist:** Follow with a Seated Twist to improve digestion and spinal flexibility. Inhale as you lengthen your spine, then exhale as you twist to the right, placing your left hand on your right thigh and your right hand on the back of the chair. Hold for a few breaths and switch sides.

6. **Seated Warrior Pose:** Transition to Seated Warrior Pose for balance and core engagement. Hold each side for several breaths, extending your

arms overhead to energize your
body.

7. **Seated Sun Salutation:**
Perform a modified version of
Sun Salutation, incorporating
seated variations of the classic
sequence to enhance your
flexibility and circulation. Flow
through this sequence a few
times:

- Inhale, raise your arms
  overhead.

- Exhale, bring your hands
  to your heart center.

- Inhale, reach your arms
  up again.

- Exhale, fold forward.

- Inhale, lift your chest
  halfway.

- Exhale, fold forward again.

- Inhale, raise your arms overhead.

- Exhale, return your hands to your heart center.

8. **Final Relaxation (Savasana):** Finish your morning sequence with a short relaxation period in your chair. Close your eyes, take a few deep breaths, and let go of any tension.

4.2 Chair Yoga for Stress Relief

This Chair Yoga sequence is tailored to help reduce stress and promote relaxation. It incorporates gentle stretches, deep breathing, and mindfulness techniques to calm the mind and ease tension.

1. **Seated Mountain Pose (Centering):** Begin with Seated Mountain Pose, focusing on grounding and centering yourself through deep, mindful breathing.

2. **Deep Belly Breathing:** Sit comfortably and place one hand on your chest and the other on your abdomen. Take slow, deep breaths, focusing on expanding your abdomen as you inhale and contracting it as you exhale. Continue for several minutes.

3. **Seated Cat-Cow Stretch:** Flow between Seated Cat and Cow stretches to release tension

in the back and encourage relaxation. Perform this sequence for a few minutes, coordinating your breath with the movements.

4. **Seated Forward Bend with Deep Breathing:** Perform the Seated Forward Bend while incorporating deep, rhythmic breaths. Inhale as you lengthen your spine, and exhale as you fold forward. Feel the breath relax your body as you hold the stretch for several breaths.

5. **Alternate Nostril Breathing (Nadi Shodhana):** Sit comfortably, spine straight. Use your right thumb to close off your right nostril and inhale deeply through your left nostril. Close off your left nostril with your right ring finger, release

your right nostril, and exhale through it. Inhale through the right nostril, close it, release the left nostril, and exhale through the left. Continue this pattern for several rounds.

6. **Seated Relaxation (Savasana):** Finish the sequence with a period of relaxation in your chair. Close your eyes, let go of any tension, and focus on your breath and the sensations in your body.

These Chair Yoga sequences can be adapted to your needs and performed at your own pace. Whether you're looking to start your day with energy or find relief from stress, these sequences offer accessible and effective practices to enhance your overall well-being.

4.3 Chair Yoga for Better Posture

This Chair Yoga sequence is designed to improve posture by strengthening the core muscles and promoting awareness of body alignment. Maintaining good posture not only enhances physical well-being but also contributes to increased confidence and overall body awareness.

1. **Seated Mountain Pose (Centering):** Begin with Seated Mountain Pose to ground yourself and establish a strong foundation for good posture. Focus on aligning your spine and maintaining an upright position.

2. **Seated Cat-Cow Stretch:** Flow through Seated Cat-Cow stretches to release tension in

the spine and create flexibility
in the back. This movement
encourages awareness of your
spinal alignment.

3. **Seated Backbend:** Sit up
   straight and place your hands
   on your lower back for support.
   Gently arch your spine, lifting
   your chest and looking upward
   while keeping your feet firmly
   on the ground. Hold for a few
   breaths, emphasizing the
   extension of your upper back.

4. **Seated Forward Bend:**
   Transition into Seated Forward
   Bend to stretch and lengthen
   your spine. Focus on
   maintaining a straight back as
   you reach toward your feet.
   Hold the pose for several
   breaths.

5. **Seated Twist:** Perform Seated Twist poses to increase spinal mobility and strengthen the core muscles responsible for maintaining good posture. Twist to the right and then to the left, holding each side for a few breaths.

6. **Seated Warrior Pose:** Practice Seated Warrior Pose to improve balance and engage the core muscles. Hold each side for a few breaths, emphasizing the strength and stability of your core.

7. **Shoulder Rolls:** Sit tall and roll your shoulders backward in a circular motion for several rounds. This movement helps release tension in the shoulders and upper back, key areas for maintaining good posture.

8. **Seated Mountain Pose with Breath Awareness:** Return to Seated Mountain Pose, focusing on your breath and the alignment of your spine. Inhale deeply, feeling your spine lengthen, and exhale, engaging your core muscles to support your posture.

9. **Final Relaxation (Savasana):** End your posture-focused Chair Yoga sequence with a brief relaxation period. Close your eyes, take a few deep breaths, and allow yourself to release any remaining tension.

4.4 Chair Yoga for Flexibility

This Chair Yoga sequence focuses on increasing flexibility throughout the body, with an emphasis on gentle stretching and mindful movement.

1. **Seated Mountain Pose (Centering):** Begin with Seated Mountain Pose to center yourself and prepare for a flexible practice. Take a few deep breaths to settle into your body.

2. **Seated Cat-Cow Stretch:** Flow through Seated Cat-Cow stretches to release tension in the spine and promote flexibility in the back. Coordinate your breath with the movements to enhance the stretch.

3. **Seated Forward Bend:**
   Perform Seated Forward Bend
   to stretch the hamstrings and
   lower back. Focus on reaching
   as far as is comfortable while
   maintaining proper alignment.
   Hold the pose for several
   breaths.

4. **Seated Side Stretch:** Gently
   stretch the sides of your body
   with Seated Side Stretches.
   Inhale as you lift your right arm
   overhead and exhale as you
   bend to the left, creating a
   lateral stretch. Repeat on the
   other side, holding each stretch
   for a few breaths.

5. **Seated Butterfly Stretch:**
   Bring the soles of your feet
   together, allowing your knees
   to fall outward. Hold your feet
   with your hands and gently

press your knees toward the floor. Hold the stretch for several breaths to open the hips and inner thighs.

6. **Seated Wide-Legged Forward Bend:** Extend your legs wide apart. Inhale as you lengthen your spine, and exhale as you fold forward from the hips. Hold this stretch for a few breaths, feeling the stretch in your inner thighs and hamstrings.

7. **Seated Twist:** Perform Seated Twists to improve spinal mobility and promote flexibility in the torso. Twist to the right and then to the left, holding each side for a few breaths.

8. **Seated Hip Flexor Stretch:** Sit up tall and extend your right leg straight while keeping your left foot flat on the floor. Inhale to lengthen your spine, and exhale as you hinge forward from your hips, reaching for your right toes. Hold for several breaths and switch sides.

9. **Final Relaxation (Savasana):** Conclude your flexibility-focused Chair Yoga sequence with a brief relaxation in your chair. Close your eyes, take a few deep breaths, and let go of any lingering tension in your body.

These Chair Yoga sequences for better posture and flexibility can be customized to your preferences and needs. Regular practice of these sequences can lead to increased body awareness, improved posture, and enhanced flexibility, contributing to your overall physical well-being.

CHAPTER 5

Breathing and Meditation Techniques

5.1 Chair Yoga Breathing Exercises

Chair Yoga breathing exercises are a vital component of this practice, helping to promote relaxation, reduce stress, and enhance mindfulness. Here are a few chair-based breathing exercises you can incorporate into your routine:

1. Deep Belly Breathing:

- Sit comfortably in your chair with your feet flat on the floor and your hands resting on your thighs.

- Close your eyes if it feels comfortable.

- Inhale deeply through your nose, allowing your abdomen to expand fully as you fill your lungs.

- Exhale slowly and completely through your nose, feeling your abdomen gently contract.

- Focus on the rise and fall of your abdomen as you breathe deeply and rhythmically.

- Continue for several minutes, letting go of tension with each exhalation.

2. 4-7-8 Breathing:

- Sit comfortably with your back straight.

- Close your eyes if you prefer.

- Inhale quietly through your nose to a mental count of four.

- Hold your breath for a count of seven.

- Exhale completely and audibly through your mouth for a count of eight.

- Repeat this cycle for several rounds, gradually extending the counts if comfortable.

3. Alternate Nostril Breathing (Nadi Shodhana):

- Sit comfortably with your spine straight and shoulders relaxed.

- Use your right thumb to close your right nostril and inhale through your left nostril.

- Close your left nostril with your right ring finger, release your right nostril, and exhale through it.

- Inhale through your right nostril, then close it, release your left nostril, and exhale through the left.

- Continue this alternating pattern for several minutes, focusing on your breath and finding a sense of balance and calm.

5.2 Mindfulness Meditation in a Chair

Mindfulness meditation can be practiced effectively while seated in a chair, making it accessible to individuals of various physical abilities. Here's a guide to practicing mindfulness meditation in a chair:

1. Find a Comfortable Seated Position:

- Sit upright in a chair with your feet flat on the floor and your hands resting on your thighs.

- Rest your hands palms up or palms down, whatever feels more comfortable to you.

- Close your eyes gently if you're comfortable doing so, or keep them slightly open with a soft gaze.

2. Focus on Your Breath:

- Bring your attention to your breath. Notice the sensation of your breath as it flows in and out of your nostrils or the gentle rise and fall of your abdomen with each breath.

3. Be Present:

- Your mind may wander, and thoughts may arise. When this happens, acknowledge the thought without judgment, and gently bring your focus back to your breath.

- Notice any physical sensations, sounds, or emotions without attachment or judgment. Let them come and go like passing clouds.

4. Set a Timer:

- If you're new to meditation, start with a shorter duration, like 5-10 minutes. Gradually increase the time as you become more comfortable with the practice.

5. Conclude Mindfully:

- When your meditation session is over, take a few deep breaths.

- Slowly open your eyes if they were closed.

- Take a moment to appreciate the benefits of your practice and carry this sense of mindfulness into your daily activities.

Mindfulness meditation in a chair offers you a valuable opportunity to cultivate awareness, reduce stress, and enhance mental clarity and relaxation.

With regular practice, you can experience increased mindfulness and a greater sense of inner peace and well-being.

CHAPTER 6

Chair Yoga for Special Populations

Chair Yoga is a versatile practice that can be adapted to meet the needs of various special populations, including seniors and individuals with disabilities. It offers the benefits of yoga while providing support and accessibility.

6.1 Chair Yoga for Seniors

Chair Yoga for seniors is a gentle and effective way to promote physical and mental well-being while considering the unique needs and limitations that can come with age. It focuses on maintaining and improving mobility, flexibility, balance, and mental clarity.

Key considerations for Chair Yoga for Seniors:

1. **Gentle Movements:** Emphasize slow, controlled movements that are easy on the joints and muscles. Avoid sudden or strenuous poses.

2. **Seated Poses:** Most poses should be done while seated in a stable chair to ensure safety and comfort.

3. **Breathing Exercises:** Incorporate simple breathing exercises to reduce stress, improve lung capacity, and increase oxygen flow.

4. **Chair Support:** Use the chair for balance and support during standing poses, ensuring it's stable and placed on a non-slip surface.

5. **Adaptations:** Be prepared to offer adaptations and modifications for individuals with varying abilities and mobility levels.

6. **Mindfulness and Relaxation:** Include mindfulness meditation and relaxation techniques to promote mental clarity, reduce anxiety, and enhance overall well-being.

6.2 Chair Yoga for Individuals with Disabilities

Chair Yoga for individuals with disabilities is a highly adaptable practice that can cater to a wide range of needs and abilities. It can be a powerful tool for improving physical function, increasing body awareness, and promoting relaxation.

Key considerations for Chair Yoga for Individuals with Disabilities:

1. **Individualized Approach:** Tailor the practice to the specific needs and abilities of each participant. Take into account any physical, sensory, or cognitive disabilities.

2. **Accessible Poses:** Choose poses that are appropriate for

the individual's mobility and flexibility. Focus on poses that can be safely done in a seated position.

3. **Chair Variations:** Consider using different types of chairs (e.g., wheelchairs, specialized adaptive chairs) to accommodate the individual's needs.

4. **Assistive Devices:** Be open to the use of assistive devices such as straps, blocks, or cushions to provide additional support and comfort.

5. **Communication:** Ensure clear communication with participants to understand their preferences, limitations, and any modifications needed.

6. **Patience and Compassion:**
   Approach the practice with
   patience and compassion,
   recognizing that progress may
   be gradual and that the primary
   goal is to promote well-being.

7. **Emphasis on Breath:** Place
   emphasis on the breath and
   mindful awareness to help
   participants connect with their
   bodies and reduce stress.

8. **Inclusivity:** Create an inclusive
   and supportive environment
   that encourages participants to
   explore their abilities and
   engage with the practice at their
   own pace.

Both Chair Yoga for seniors and
Chair Yoga for individuals with
disabilities can be adapted and
customized to provide physical,

mental, and emotional benefits to these special populations. The key is to prioritize safety, accessibility, and individualized instruction to ensure a positive and empowering experience for all participants.

6.3 Chair Yoga for Office Workers

Office workers often spend extended periods sitting at desks, which can lead to physical discomfort, tension, and reduced productivity. Chair Yoga for office workers is an excellent way to counter these challenges and promote physical and mental well-being without leaving the office environment. Here's a tailored approach:

Key considerations for Chair Yoga for Office Workers:

1. **Office-Friendly Poses:** Select poses and stretches that can be comfortably and discreetly performed at a desk or in a chair. These should not require getting on the floor or extensive space.

2. **Regular Breaks:** Encourage office workers to take short breaks throughout the day to perform Chair Yoga exercises. These breaks can boost energy and alleviate stiffness.

3. **Breathing Techniques:** Incorporate quick, effective breathing exercises to reduce stress and increase mental clarity during the workday.

4. **Seated Poses:** Focus on seated poses and stretches that target common areas of tension for office workers, such as the neck, shoulders, wrists, and lower back.

5. **Mindfulness Breaks:** Encourage brief mindfulness breaks where employees can center themselves, reduce stress, and regain focus.

6. **Chair Support:** Ensure that the chair being used is stable and comfortable. If needed, provide guidance on proper chair ergonomics.

7. **Adjustable Sequences:** Tailor Chair Yoga sequences to accommodate varying levels of flexibility and mobility among office workers.

Sample Chair Yoga Sequence for Office Workers:

Perform each of these poses for a few breaths and repeat the sequence as needed during the workday.

1. **Seated Mountain Pose:** Sit up straight with your feet flat on the floor. Inhale and reach your arms overhead, stretching upward. Exhale and bring your hands back to your lap.

2. **Neck Rolls:** Gently roll your head to the right, chin to chest, and then to the left, creating a circular motion. Reverse the direction after a few rolls.

3. **Shoulder Shrugs:** Inhale, shrug your shoulders up toward your ears, and exhale as you release them down. Repeat a few times.

4. **Wrist Flexor Stretch:** Extend your right arm straight with the palm facing down. Use your left hand to gently pull your right fingers back. Hold for a few breaths and switch sides.

5. **Seated Cat-Cow Stretch:** Sit at the edge of your chair and inhale as you arch your back (Cow) and exhale as you round your back (Cat). Repeat a few times.

6. **Seated Forward Bend:** Sit back in your chair and inhale as you lengthen your spine. Exhale as you hinge at your hips and reach your hands toward your toes or the floor. Hold for a few breaths.

7. **Desk Yoga:** Use your desk for support by placing your hands

on it, then step back and create a straight line from your hands to your hips, stretching your back and legs.

8. **Desk Neck Stretch:** Sit or stand, place your left hand on the right side of your head, and gently tilt your head toward your left shoulder. Hold for a few breaths and switch sides.

9. **Mindfulness Break:** Close your eyes, take several deep breaths, and bring your awareness to your breath. Focus on the sensation of each inhale and exhale for a minute.

Chair Yoga for office workers can be a valuable addition to the workday, promoting physical comfort, mental clarity, and overall well-being, all within the confines of the office environment. Encourage employees to incorporate these practices into their daily routine to reap the benefits of Chair Yoga at work.

CHAPTER 7

Tips for Progression and Challenges

7.1 Gradually Increasing Intensity

Progression in yoga, including Chair Yoga, is essential for continued growth and development. Gradually increasing the intensity of your Chair Yoga practice can help you gain strength, flexibility, and mindfulness. Here are some tips for achieving this progression:

1. Consistent Practice: The foundation of progression is consistent practice. Dedicate a specific time each day or week for your Chair Yoga practice. Regularity allows you to build upon previous sessions.

2. Mindful Awareness: Pay close attention to your body and its responses during each practice. Mindful awareness helps you gauge your limits and determine when it's appropriate to intensify your practice.

3. Breath Awareness: Sync your breath with your movements. As you become more comfortable with the basics, try to extend your inhales and exhales, promoting better breath control and mindfulness.

4. Explore Variations: Begin with the fundamental Chair Yoga poses and gradually explore more advanced variations. For example, if you're comfortable with Seated Forward

Bend, you can add a twist or reach further with each practice session.

5. Hold Poses Longer: Increase the duration you hold poses. Start with a few breaths and gradually work up to holding poses for a minute or longer. Longer holds promote strength and flexibility.

6. Add Sequences: Progress from individual poses to sequences. Combine poses to create flowing sequences that challenge your body and mind. For instance, you can link Seated Mountain Pose, Seated Forward Bend, and Seated Twist into a flowing sequence.

7. Incorporate Resistance: To increase strength, consider incorporating light resistance into your practice. You can use resistance bands or small weights during seated exercises to add a strength-training component.

8. Explore Balance Poses: Once you're comfortable with seated poses, experiment with balance poses. Lift one foot off the floor or try poses like Seated Tree Pose to challenge your stability.

9. Practice Mindfulness Meditation: Introduce mindfulness meditation to your practice. Meditating regularly can deepen your awareness and enhance your overall well-being.

10. Attend Classes or Workshops: Consider attending Chair Yoga classes or workshops led by experienced instructors. They can provide guidance on progression and offer new challenges tailored to your level.

11. Listen to Your Body: The most important tip is to listen to your body. If you experience pain or discomfort, back off from the intensity and focus on maintaining proper form and alignment. Pushing too hard can lead to injury.

12. Patience and Self-Compassion: Understand that progression in yoga is a journey, and it's different for everyone. Be patient with yourself and practice self-compassion. Celebrate your achievements and acknowledge your efforts.

13. Seek Guidance: If you have specific goals or challenges, consider seeking guidance from a qualified yoga instructor or physical therapist. They can provide personalized guidance and modifications to address your needs.

Progression in Chair Yoga is not about competition or pushing yourself beyond your limits. It's about gradual growth, mindful exploration, and self-improvement. By following these tips and honoring your body's capabilities and limitations, you can experience the many benefits of Chair Yoga while progressing at your own pace.

7.2 Incorporating Props

Incorporating props into your Chair Yoga practice can enhance your experience, provide support, and help you deepen your practice. Props can be especially beneficial for individuals with limited flexibility or mobility. Here are some tips on how to incorporate props effectively into your Chair Yoga practice:

1. Chair Variations: Start with the chair itself. Chairs come in various shapes and sizes, and you can choose one that suits your needs. Consider using a stable chair with a high backrest for added support during seated poses.

2. Cushions or Pillows: Placing cushions or pillows on your chair can provide added comfort and support, especially for seated poses. You can use them to raise the height of the seat or cushion your back.

3. Yoga Blocks: Yoga blocks are versatile props that can be used in Chair Yoga to modify poses and make them more accessible. For example:

- Place a block under your feet to raise them during seated poses.

- Use blocks as armrests to support your arms during balancing poses.

- Sit on a block to raise your hips and improve alignment in seated poses.

4. Resistance Bands: Resistance bands can add an element of strength training to your Chair Yoga practice. You can incorporate them into exercises to increase resistance and build muscle strength.

5. Yoga Straps: Yoga straps can be useful for extending your reach in seated stretches. They are particularly helpful for individuals with limited flexibility.

6. Blankets: Folded blankets can provide extra cushioning and support when placed on the seat or backrest of the chair. They can also be used for padding under the knees during certain poses.

7. Neck Support: If you have neck issues, consider using a small rolled-up towel or neck pillow to support your neck during seated and reclined poses.

8. Eye Pillow: For relaxation and meditation, use an eye pillow to cover your eyes and block out light. This can enhance your sense of calm and help you focus inward.

9. Bolsters: While not commonly used in Chair Yoga, bolsters can be placed on the seat of the chair to provide added cushioning and support for seated poses.

10. Blanket Rolls: Roll up a blanket and place it behind your lower back for added lumbar support during seated poses. This can be especially helpful if you have lower back discomfort.

11. Wall Support: If your practice space allows, practice Chair Yoga near a wall. You can use the wall for balance and support during standing poses or as a reference point for alignment.

12. Personalize Your Props: Adapt your props to your specific needs. Experiment with different combinations of props to find what works best for your body and practice.

13. Instructor Guidance: If you're new to using props or unsure about how to incorporate them effectively, consider taking a Chair Yoga class or working with an experienced instructor. They can provide guidance and modifications tailored to your needs.

Remember that props are tools to assist and support your practice, not crutches. They should enhance your experience and help you access poses more comfortably and safely. Feel free to explore and experiment with different props to find what works best for you in your Chair Yoga practice.

7.3 Overcoming Common Challenges

Chair Yoga is a versatile and accessible practice, but like any form of yoga, it can come with its own set of challenges. Here are some common challenges that people may encounter in Chair Yoga and tips on how to overcome them:

1. Limited Mobility:

- **Challenge:** Limited mobility can make it difficult to perform some poses or transitions.

- **Solution:** Focus on poses that are comfortable and attainable for your range of motion. Gradually work on improving mobility with gentle stretches and regular practice.

2. Balance Issues:

- **Challenge:** Balance can be a concern, especially for seniors or individuals with balance issues.

- **Solution:** Use the chair for support during balance poses. Hold onto the backrest or armrests as needed. Over time, your balance may improve with practice.

3. Pain or Discomfort:

- **Challenge:** Pain or discomfort, particularly in the lower back or neck, can deter people from practicing regularly.

- **Solution:** Pay attention to proper alignment in poses and use props, such as cushions or folded blankets, for added support. If you experience pain, modify or skip poses that exacerbate it.

4. Lack of Focus:

- **Challenge:** It can be challenging to maintain focus and mindfulness during practice, especially for beginners.

- **Solution:** Practice mindfulness techniques, such as breath awareness, to help improve concentration. Set an intention for your practice to stay present and relaxed.

5. Feeling Self-Conscious:

- **Challenge:** Some individuals may feel self-conscious about practicing Chair Yoga in a group setting.

- **Solution:** Remember that Chair Yoga is for everyone, and there's no judgment in the practice. If self-consciousness is a concern, consider practicing at home initially until you feel more comfortable.

6. Adapting Poses:

- **Challenge:** Adapting poses to individual needs can be

challenging, especially without guidance.

- **Solution:** Seek guidance from a qualified Chair Yoga instructor who can provide modifications and adjustments tailored to your specific challenges and goals.

7. Patience:

- **Challenge:** Progress in Chair Yoga may be slower than expected, and impatience can be a barrier.

- **Solution:** Understand that yoga is a journey, and it's essential to be patient with yourself. Celebrate small achievements along the way, and don't rush the process.

8. Finding Time:

- **Challenge:** Finding time for regular practice in a busy schedule can be difficult.

- **Solution:** Schedule your Chair Yoga practice into your daily or weekly routine, even if it's just for a few minutes at a time. Consistency is key to seeing progress.

9. Avoiding Overexertion:

- **Challenge:** Some individuals may push themselves too hard, leading to overexertion or injury.

- **Solution:** Listen to your body and practice within your comfort zone. Yoga is about self-care, not pushing your limits. Avoid forcing yourself into poses that don't feel right.

10. Motivation:

- **Challenge:** Staying motivated to practice regularly can be tough.

- **Solution:** Set achievable goals and rewards for yourself. Connect with a community of Chair Yoga practitioners for support and encouragement. Remind yourself of the physical and mental benefits you experience after each session.

Chair Yoga is adaptable, and you can tailor it to your specific needs and challenges. By addressing these common obstacles with patience, self-compassion, and a willingness to adapt, you can overcome them and enjoy the many benefits of Chair Yoga.

www.ingramcontent.com/pod-product-compliance
Lightning Source LLC
Chambersburg PA
CBHW050835260726
48660CB00006B/2248